Hidden Dangers

The Truth About Seed Oils and Their Impact on Our Health

Olivia Phillips

© **Copyright 2022 - All rights reserved.**

The content contained within this book may not be reproduced, duplicated or transmitted without direct written permission from the author or the publisher.

Under no circumstances will any blame or legal responsibility be held against the publisher, or author, for any damages, reparation, or monetary loss due to the information contained within this book, either directly or indirectly.

Legal Notice:

This book is copyright protected. It is only for personal use. You cannot amend, distribute, sell, use, quote or paraphrase any part, or the content within this book, without the consent of the author or publisher.

Disclaimer Notice:

Please note the information contained within this document is for educational and entertainment purposes only. All effort has been executed to present accurate, up to date, reliable, complete information. No warranties of any kind are declared or implied. Readers acknowledge that the author is not engaged in the rendering of legal, financial, medical or professional advice. The content within this book has been derived from various sources. Please consult a licensed professional before attempting any techniques outlined in this book.

By reading this document, the reader agrees that under no circumstances is the author responsible for any losses, direct or indirect, that are incurred as a result of the use of the information contained within this document, including, but not limited to, errors, omissions, or inaccuracies.

Scan this QR code for free future books, free audible codes (when available), and to learn when all of my newest books are released!

Contents

Introduction	vii
1. The History of Seed Oils	1
2. The Science of Seed Oils	6
3. Hidden Dangers of Popular Seed Oils	12
4. Healthy Alternatives to Seed Oils	21
Conclusion	41
Bibliography	45

Introduction

You've certainly heard of seed oils, but what are they and where do they come from? First of all, "seed oils" is a general term for a large array of refined oils that come from diverse vegetables. Some of these include sunflower, soybean, canola, and grapeseed oils. However, unlike other vegetable-based oils that are not considered seed oils, such as olive oil, seed oils are usually prepared through a synthetic chemistry extraction system that may include other processes such as bleaching.

The prevalence of seed oils in the food industry and, by consequence, in the food we eat is enormous. Seed oils are not only a recurring ingredient when we cook, but they can also be found in most processed foods that, besides having preservatives and additives, also contain industrial seed oils.

Now, seed oils have many negative impacts on our health, mostly because they are inflammatory to the body, have almost no nutrients, are high in calories, and are hard to

Introduction

digest. The consequences of using seed oils don't end here, and we explore more through this book. In fact, that is exactly the goal of this book: to expose the overall hidden dangers of seed oils for our health and how they affect obesity and chronic diseases.

Chapter 1
The History of Seed Oils

Any food that comes to the market today has to go through an array of tests, clinical trials, and many other checks before it can be sold to the public. In fact, not only food has to go through such a thorough process, but other types of products, such as drugs, also have to undergo rigorous checks before they reach humans. Throughout all of these checks and tests, we have safety experts and regulators that analyze all the procedures to make sure everything is safe to consume. We can say that most foods or drugs that are sold to the public are safe, even if there are still some exceptions where certain products had to be taken off the market because of issues that were not identified throughout the tests and trials.

This wasn't exactly the case when the first mass-market seed oil, which was a hydrogenated oil, was brought to the shelves. The name for this oil is Crisco, which can still be found in most supermarkets today, even if it started production back in the early 1900s. However, this wasn't the first seed oil to slip into our modern diet; that was in the late 1800s, although these weren't mass-produced.

Even back then, seed oils had critics among the academic community, mostly because of the lack of regulation in the food industry. To give you an idea, the very first consumer protection law was passed in 1906, but even then, it wasn't a law to look into the safety of seed oils or other food products, but simply to label all products accurately, which seed oils were. With this, what we are trying to say is that when seed oils came into our modern diet, there were little to no regulations. Only in 1938 was the Federal Food, Drug, and Cosmetic Act written. However, with that act, a list of "generally recognized as safe" (GRAS) products was created, which stated that widespread use of products before 1958 would fall into the GRAS list and not be tested, and only new products coming onto the market would have to be tested and trialed. Most seed oils were widespread way before the FDA act was written in 1958; for instance, corn oil started to be used around 1898, peanut oil around the 1930s, and safflower oil around the 1940s. There was an exception for canola oil, which started to be mass-produced around 1974, but it only underwent allergen tests, chemical composition tests, and fatty acid profile tests, which are still important tests to make, but they are not sufficient to be deemed proper for human consumption.

But if seed oils had a bad reputation given by the likes of reputable magazines such as "Popular Science," how did they become such an essential ingredient in most western cuisine? Well, that has to do with, again, the first mass-produced seed oil, Crisco. For many years since its mass production began, Crisco had a single ingredient: cottonseed oil, although because the Federal Food, Drug, and Cosmetic Act only came into being in 1938, most people were unaware of what it contained. And due to the geniality of Crisco's marketers, who advertised their product as a healthier alternative than saturated animal fats, Crisco's brand grew exponentially. But before we go into how they made that happen, let's first understand why cottonseed oil came to be and what techniques made it possible.

During the 19th century, cotton seeds were an inconvenience, mostly because when used to create fiber for clothing, they left behind an immeasurable amount of seeds that farmers tried to transform into oil, but it wasn't very commercially viable because of its dark color and pungent smell. However, David Wesson, a chemist who came up with the deodorizing and bleaching techniques used on cottonseed oil, made possible the neutralization of the strong smell and also the clearing of the dark oil, which gave it much more commercial potential. It wasn't long until cottonseed oil started to be mixed with other animal fats to make it cheaper.

The rival for cottonseed oil was lard, which had been produced at home for much longer now, and during the late 19th century, it started to be mass-produced. However, even though it had a very strong pig taste to it, that wasn't the biggest issue with lard; its cost was. This is where cottonseed oil companies saw an opportunity. Cottonseed oil producers had to change people's opinions about their product if they were to compete with lard, since cotton was just associated with clothes, not food. In fact, early cottonseed producers didn't think that was an issue, and they often highlighted the connection with the textile industry.

However, in 1911, Crisco was established, and they were able to see the bigger problem and make significant changes when it came to advertising their product. It was not that Crisco's product was that different from the likes of Cotosuet or Cottolene (early producers of cottonseed); it was pretty much the same, but instead of mixing cottonseed with fat, they used a newly discovered procedure called "hydrogenation." This was essentially a chemical procedure where two hydrogen atoms were added to fatty acids, which allowed a certain plasticity and firmness to the shortenings. This allowed the consistency of Crisco's product to be slightly different. Another major difference we can clearly see just by looking at their names is the omission of the word "cotton" in Crisco's name. These two differences, as well as the omission of cottonseed in the process of creating the product, made the public believe this was an entirely new product. Remember that at the time, companies didn't need to mention the ingredients in their products. While most products on the market did have a list of ingredients on their labels, Crisco's marketing team decided to advertise the product without mentioning exactly what Crisco was. In their own words, through advertising, they mentioned that Crisco was made of 100% shortening, or that it was all vegetable and made from vegetable oil, or sometimes using the slogan "Crisco is Crisco, and nothing else."

The main reason for this marketing change from Crisco was that cottonseed didn't have the best reputation when they launched their product because of some companies that used cheap cottonseed to produce cheaper olive oil, but also because of the link between cottonseed oil and dyes in the textile industry. So, Crisco chose to focus on a total rebrand and leave out cottonseed as an ingredient in their advertisements. Because of this change, Crisco started selling well as soon as it was launched since it was better for frying than olive oil, didn't have the smell lard had, and had a longer shelf life than other ingredients used to fry, such as butter. From there, Crisco just grew in popularity.

While today Crisco doesn't use cottonseed, replacing it with canola, soy, or palm oil, it's still used across the country, such as a main ingredient in processed foods or to fry. It was its ingenious marketing capabilities that allowed Crisco to become an extremely popular brand, and even when the government created the Pure Food and Drug Act, which demanded all food and pharmaceutical companies to list all the ingredients and components in their products' labels, Crisco managed to avoid doing that by stating that trusted brands didn't need consumers to know or understand what ingredients were in processed food. This is still widely used for many products today, such as Cheetos or Spam.

Chapter 2
The Science of Seed Oils

One of the main differences between seed oils and traditional fats is that, while they are both mixtures of triglycerides, oils are liquid at room temperature, such as sunflower oil, while fats are solid, such as lard. Another big difference is that solid fats come from animals, while oils come from plants and fish. There are some exceptions, such as palm or coconut oils, which are solid at room temperature due to their high content of saturated fatty acids. However, both oils and fats are composed of a mix of unsaturated and saturated fatty acids. While solid fats have more saturated fats, which lead to a higher risk of heart problems, oils also have an excessive amount that is not healthy for your body.

From a scientific point of view, the average composition of most seed oils has about 57.85% fat, 10.07% carbohydrates, 26.39% proteins, 3.61% moisture, and 2.08% ash (Ouilly et al., 2017).

The Impact of Seed Oils on Inflammation, Cardiovascular Health, and Chronic Diseases

Besides the lack of regulation when it comes to seed oils, it's relatively well-known that these ingredients that we often use to cook also have vast consequences for our health, in particular on bodily inflammation and cardiovascular health, due to some of the components they have.

According to a recent study, due to the consumption of seed oils in our diet, the average person can have about 30% polyunsaturated fat when a healthy person should only have about 2% (Nast, 2021). And this is caused by the high concentration of these types of components in seed oils. In turn, this increases the chances of development of body inflammation, which can contribute to many other issues such as heart disease, obesity, and even diabetes. However, this excess of polyunsaturated fat is not the only component that puts our lives at risk. Because of the many chemical processes in seed oils, they also have a high concentration of omega-6 fatty acids, which only increase bodily inflammation more. This destabilizes the balance between our body's omega-3 and omega-6 fatty acids, leading to these types of chronic diseases. In sum, it's this unbalance of omega-3 and omega-6 fatty acids that causes the western world to have so many cases of obesity and chronic diseases.

The main reason most people in the western world still choose to use seed oils to cook is because of years of faulty research funded by seed oil companies. Most of the conclusions reached by those researchers determined that seed oils were actually "heart healthy" because of their low concentration of LDL cholesterol, but that doesn't prevent the development of inflammatory diseases. As we've seen, it is the fatty acids that provoke those issues. As a result, it is one of the primary causes of a large obese population.

Seed oils are also largely responsible for chronic cardiovascular diseases. It all starts throughout the process of refining the oil, when certain amounts of trans fat are created from the unsaturated fats. However, when you use seed oil for frying, these are also created. Now, we've had many researchers point out that trans fat increases blood cholesterol by causing bodily inflammation and, with that, cardiovascular issues (Oteng & Kersten, 2019). Some studies also compare the consumption of trans fats before 1911 (when Procter & Gamble came up with the partially hydrogenated process to create Crisco) and today. As we've mentioned, most trans fats in seed oils are formed throughout the chemical process that most vegetable oils undergo, but they were also found in snacks and some baked goods until they were banned in 2018.

We've talked about saturated fats and trans fats, but there's another type of fat in seed oils that also has consequences for your body—oxidized fats. Most seed oils go rancid or putrid after some time in your cupboard, and this happens because polyunsaturated fats such as omega-3 and omega-6, when in contact with heat and oxygen, oxidize. This doesn't exclusively happen on the shelf, but also in the frying pan and in your body. These cause inflammation too, clogging your arteries and creating cardiovascular problems.

Hidden Dangers

From an evolutionary point of view, seed oils are a mismatch, and this makes them the main culprit in chronic diseases nowadays. This is all due to the excessive amounts of some of the components we've talked about that go against our past ancestry and create in us all of these types of health issues.

Industrially created seed oils have, among many other components, an excess of calories. Up until the creation of industrial seed oils around the 1900s, no human was even consuming much or any type of seed oil. However, since the 1970s, we've seen an exponential increase in the consumption of all types of seed oils. To give you an idea, this increased seed oil consumption per person in a year from 3 or 4 pounds to 26 pounds in a single year (Blasbalg et al., 2011). The main fatty acid in seed oils is linoleic acid, which today accounts for about 8% of all the calories we consume. If we compare this to our ancestors when they were hunters and gatherers, such acid accounted for only about 1%–2% of their diets (Ramsden et al., 2009). This drastic change, for which our bodies were not prepared, is the number-one cause responsible for chronic diseases.

These are also high in additives, which contribute to people's poor health. Seed oil companies, in an attempt to prolong the shelf life of their products, add synthetic antioxidants. These antioxidants are predominantly TBHQ, BHT, and BHA and have immune-disrupting, endocrine-disrupting, and carcinogenic effects (Nobuyuki Ito et al., 2020). TBHQ is also known to decrease the speed at which antibodies react as well as increase immunoglobulin E, which can increase the development of allergies through food. Not only that, but most seed oils come from the most genetically modified plants in the world, such as rapeseed, corn, cotton, or soy. So, not only are they full of harmful antioxidants and unhealthy fats, but most of these come from highly genetically modified plants, and even though there are only a few studies on the long-term effects of genetic modification on our health, the ones we have point out the increase in unhealthy individuals. And if none of this is enough to steer you away from seed oils, the repeated heating of seed oils, as is often done in restaurants and even at home, makes these products even more toxic than they already are. The more you heat the seed oil, the more depleted of vitamin E it becomes, and because this vitamin is a natural antioxidant, this leads to the creation of free radicals that harm your body. This also leads to some of the issues we've mentioned, such as cardiovascular problems, as well as liver issues.

There are other studies that also seem to indicate an increase in other health issues, such as asthma and autoimmune diseases, because of the rise of omega-6 fatty acids (Wendell et al., 2014). These can also cause anxiety and depression, which are connected to cognitive decline (Berger et al., 2017). Canola oil in particular has been associated with a decrease in an individual's learning ability and memory (Lauretti & Praticò, 2017).

If all these health issues don't make you look at other options when it comes to cooking with seed oils, perhaps the fact that they derive from destructive agriculture will. They are not only harmful to humans, but also to the environment. They are considered to derive from monoculture agriculture, which drains the soil of nutrients so that with each passing year, the soil becomes less rich and the crops more vulnerable to diseases. So, as we've seen, seed oils are already almost devoid of nutrients, which makes a case for switching to a healthier alternative. We will talk about these healthier alternatives later in the book, but first, and in the following chapter, we will dig a little deeper into each seed oil from a scientific point of view and analyze studies that connect them to negative health outcomes.

Chapter 3
Hidden Dangers of Popular Seed Oils

We will now go through some of the most popular seed oils and analyze the dangers they pose to our health, specifically as backed by scientific studies and articles. We've already seen the broader consequences of seed oils in the human body, but some have different effects or are even more dangerous than others. This is what we will talk about in this chapter.

Analysis of Popular Seed Oils

Soybean Oil

Soybean oil is the most widely used seed oil in the US and is often used as cooking oil; it's also used as dressings and sauces and in many packaged foods, snacks, or baked goods (USDA, n.d.). We chose to lead with this seed oil because it accounts for 40% of the major fatty acids (omega-3 and omega-6) consumed in the US. It's also often sold as a mixed vegetable oil with other oils such as sunflower, canola, or safflower oil.

When looking at the potential issues soybean oil can bring, we have to highlight the effects of saturated fats and polyunsaturated fats. While some studies have failed to find a correlation between this specific oil and coronary heart disease, most of them don't take into account the macronutrients used to replace saturated fats, which is what leads many experts to believe there is an association between the issue and the consumption of soybean oil (Messina et al., 2021). However, there have been many studies confirming the imbalance between omega-6 and omega-3 when consuming soybean oil. These fatty acids often lead to pro-oxidative states and bodily inflammation.

Health authorities in the US have been battling an obesity epidemic in the last few decades, and because of that, many studies have been conducted by researchers to find the potential cause for it. As soybean oil constitutes the main seed oil in terms of consumption in the country, we've analyzed research to find out if there is any correlation. When looking at soybean oil regarding other health issues such as obesity and diabetes, according to a report, this seed oil is far more obesogenic and diabetogenic than other more natural sugars, such as fructose (Deol et al., 2015). This particular research compares the effects of saturated fats against fructose and unsaturated fats when looking at a rise in obesity and diabetic diagnoses. This research was conducted on a male mouse whose diet was based on fat from soybean oil and coconut oil, and the results were mesmerizing. The research showed a rapid increase in weight but also a disposition for diabetes, insulin resistance, and glucose intolerance when compared to another mouse on a diet based on fats from just coconut oil. The use of a diet based on fructose did not reveal an increase in diabetes or obesity; however, it did lead to a fatty liver. When using soybean oil with fructose, there was an increase in kidney weight. This study concluded that a diet based on soybean oil increases obesity and diabetes and constitutes a risk to health, especially when compared to coconut oil.

Sunflower Oil

Sunflower oil is widely used in food, especially fried food since it doesn't have a lot of flavor, but it's also used as a skin treatment or even as a medicine. But how much impact does this seed oil have on our health? Let's start with the nutrition information.

While sunflower oil is a good source of both vitamin K and E, if we look at the main components, a tablespoon of sunflower oil has no proteins, no fiber, no sugar, and no carbohydrates. On the other hand, the same amount has 120 calories and 78 grams of fat. So, it's widely caloric and rich in fat and offers no other nutrients (WebMD Editorial Contributors, 2022).

Sunflower oil has a high concentration of polyunsaturated fatty acids, as we've mentioned before. And while there are some studies that confirm or at least associate that with positive effects on the plasma lipid profile, there are still many doubts regarding how it affects insulin resistance and inflammation. When evaluating sunflower oil and its dangers to our bodies, the study we observed yielded interesting results. They conducted the experiment on four obese mice to understand if sunflower oil had negative or positive effects on them. The first had a simple controlled diet with no addition of sunflower oil or any other substances; the second had a high fat diet (HFD); the third had a controlled diet with polyunsaturated fatty acids; and the fourth had a HFD supplemented with polyunsaturated fatty acids. It's important to note that these polyunsaturated fatty acids were coming from sunflower oil fed to the mice, and all were given to them three times a week, while the mice on the controlled diet (including those fed a high-fat diet) were given water.

The researchers found that there were no positive effects on inflammatory markers but increased cytokine production, which has pro-inflammatory effects in the body (Masi et al., 2012). However, it's also important to note that there were improvements in the plasma lipid profile.

Canola Oil

Canola oil is the most popular seed oil in Canada. It's widely used for cooking all over the world, and it's produced from a crossbreed type of rapeseed. Much like other seed oils, canola oil goes through many different processes before reaching the consumer. It starts with the cleaning process, where pods, stems, and weed seeds are removed from the canola seeds. Then it goes to the heating and flaking process, where it's placed in machines where they extract the oil. Then it goes to the cooking process, where it is cooked and heated up several times. The flakes from the cooking process go through a few presses, where the rest of the oil is extracted. Then, it goes through the refining and processing phases, where they refine the crude oil, changing its color and taste and improving the shelf life of the product. As you can see, it goes through many different phases before it's deemed consumable.

There are many studies that highlight the health risks of canola oil. For instance, in 2018 research, scientists found that it's very likely that people who cook with canola oil will develop metabolic syndrome. This is a combination of obesity, hypertension, and diabetes (Sun et al., 2018). This study was conducted in participants aged between 25 and 34 years old of the most varied weight. Among those deemed healthy (weight-wise), first they analyzed those participants that used canola oil frequently (however, that was the only fat-related behavior they engaged in) and compared it to participants that rarely or never used canola oil. The researchers used the Metabolic Syndrome Score to register their findings, and participants who rarely or never used canola oil had a much lower score than those that used canola oil frequently (in this case, the lower the score, the healthier). Among those participants that were overweight and used canola oil for cooking, the metabolic syndrome score was much higher than that of those overweight participants that never or rarely used canola oil for cooking. This study was pretty conclusive and stated that canola oil users had a much higher chance of developing metabolic syndrome than those who did not.

In a study conducted in 2020 on yellow croaker fish to understand how canola oil affected the increase of inflammation, the results pointed to that being true with a diet consisting of more than 6%; the oil created an inflammatory response (Mu et al., 2020). This was a 12-week trial on large yellow croaker fish, where their fish-oil diet was replaced by canola oil. The researchers also saw a significant decrease in the growth of yellow croaker fish as well as an increase in lipids in the liver and muscles of the fish. In sum, the study concluded that canola oil reduced their growth and induced inflammation.

It's also been pointed out that canola oil might also be related to loss of memory. In a research study from 2017, conducted in mice over six months, two groups were fed a chow diet, with one of these groups being fed chow with added canola oil (Lauretti & Praticò, 2017). The group of mice with the added canola oil saw an increase in body weight as well as issues with working memory by reducing post-synaptic density.

Corn Oil

While corn oil has what are considered healthy elements, such as phytosterols and vitamin E, it also has a high concentration of omega-6 fats. In a study conducted on mice in 2001, the researchers reached alarming conclusions. They divided a group of mice in two, with one group being fed water with corn oil and another group being fed water with a sucrose solution. The group consuming water with corn oil increased in weight faster and put on more weight than the group with the sucrose solution (Takeda et al., 2001). However, the more alarming results were observed at the end of the study, where the group of mice fed water with corn oil presented a fatty liver as well as hepatic hypertrophy. The researchers concluded that corn oil had more severe consequences for their health than sucrose.

Palm Oil

Palm oil is the most-used seed oil in the world. It's not only used in most oils, but it's also used in sweets such as cakes, biscuits, and even margarine. It can also be found in cleaning products as well as cosmetics. In a study we evaluated from 2015, researchers analyzed the effects of palm oil on several diseases, such as obesity, cardiovascular problems, and cancer. When researchers studied animals, they discovered that palm oil reduces insulin sensitivity, causing them to gain weight (Mancini et al., 2015). However, the results on humans for both cardiovascular and cancer increase were conflicting, owing to the wide age range between subjects and the lack of attention paid to other dietary elements consumed by the subjects. Either way, even if inconclusive in some parameters, the research showed a tendency for weight gain in animals that had a palm oil-based diet.

Hydrogenated Vegetable Oil

Hydrogenated oil is the process that many oils, including seed oils, go through to become solid by adding hydrogen to them. While it's not oil, since these are solids, we thought that looking at them from a health point of view would also be important to make our point. Examples of hydrogenated oil are, for instance, shortening and baked goods such as pies and cookies.

In a study published in the American Journal of Clinical Nutrition, a team of researchers wanted to study what natural trans fats in hydrogenated oils did to our cardiovascular health. To be more specific, they looked at how these trans fatty acids contributed to sudden cardiac arrest and cardiovascular mortality. These trans fatty acids are created when the process of hydrogenation is done in vegetable oils, and there has been quite some concern over the findings, not only in the study that we will mention but in many others of the same type (Ascherio & Willett, 1997). The main concern with this is that these acids are destroyed and replaced with artificial isomers that have a similar structure. However, this decreases metabolic activity, contributing to heart diseases. These acids also increase plasma levels of low-density cholesterol and decrease high-density cholesterol, and this, by increasing blood lipid concentrations, leads to coronary heart disease, which, according to this study, led to at least 30,000 premature deaths. These findings, coupled with the lack of nutritional benefits of these acids, are an even bigger statement against a diet based on hydrogenated vegetable oils.

As you can see, there are tons of studies and evidence that point out that seed oils have a negative effect on our health. Obviously, different oils might have a more damaging effect on certain systems in our body and affect people in a different way. However, basing your diet on healthier oils instead of picking the seed oils that, in theory, do less harm will certainly lead you to a better and healthier life. This is because with these types of studies there are many variables, which, at times, makes it complicated to get conclusive answers; however, this does not mean there won't be other consequences that might be proved true later in different studies.

Choosing healthier types of fats is definitely the way to go, and that is exactly what we will be talking about in the next chapter. We will list the healthiest alternatives to seed oils you can find and back them up with studies regarding the health benefits they bring.

Chapter 4
Healthy Alternatives to Seed Oils

Fortunately, there are many healthier alternatives to seed oils out there, and they taste delicious too. We understand that it might be hard to keep up with nutritional facts about what oils might be better for you, but the ones we will present you with here have been deemed healthier for a long time, so it's unlikely there will be a change. In fact, many of them have been used for centuries, so we have a much better understanding of what they do to our bodies than the newly-created seed oils.

We've divided this chapter into four different sections. We will start by analyzing traditional fats such as butter, tallow, and ghee. Then, we will move on to oils usually considered healthier, such as coconut and olive oil. We will then compare all of these alternatives with seed oils from a nutritional point of view, and we will end the chapter with some practical tips on how you can transition from seed oils to healthier alternatives.

Overview of Traditional Fats

When we mention traditional fats, we are talking about those that, as a society, we've started using way before things like seed oils came onto the market, such as tallow, which was originally created somewhere in the Middle Ages, or butter, where the first evidence of it was found around 8,000 B.C. These were the original fats used to cook by humans, and it's important to look at them to understand how different they are from the fats we use today, even though traditional fats such as butter are still widely used.

Tallow

Tallow is a fat that comes from beef (at least most of the time, since there's also tallow that comes from mutton, hogs, or pigs, but more often as a mix). It's a fat that is solid at room temperature and has high concentrations of saturated fat, but once heated, it goes into liquid form. It's not something widely used today in western cuisine but is still used; however, you might know it as beef lard or shortening, and it's quite similar in terms of appearance and texture to butter, but it has a lighter color. Tallow is created from the fat around an animal's organs, such as the kidneys. Nutritionally speaking, and taking measures from the US Department of Agriculture, a single tablespoon of tallow has no carbs, sugar, fiber, or protein, but it has around 115 calories and 13 grams of fat (both unsaturated and saturated) (US Department of Agriculture, n.d.). As you'd suppose, grass-fed cattle produce the best quality of tallow; however, the most abundant tallow comes from cattle raised on feedlots. To give you an idea, tallow from grass-fed cattle is higher in vitamin A, D, E, and B12, as well as more CLA and choline (Levy, 2020).

Tallow has more health benefits than seed oils, but it is still considered a fat and should be consumed in moderation. This type of fat provides people with more healthy fats than those processed fats that are so abundant in western cuisine. With about 40–50% of tallow's composition made of unsaturated fats, we've previously pointed out the benefits of these types of fats to our hearts, while the saturated fats found in tallow have mostly neutral effects on our bodies, especially when compared to processed saturated fats from seed oils (Heileson, 2019). This allows the increase of what specialists call "good cholesterol," which, when consumed moderately, shouldn't raise your cardiovascular risks. While when adding seed oils to your diet, you'd be consuming the same type of fats that you would if you used tallow, the main difference here is that with tallow, you are consuming natural fats instead of processed ones.

Because tallow has a high concentration of CLA, there's research evidence that states it can be beneficial to weight loss (Whigham et al., 2007). This is because of how it interacts with the human metabolism and has the consequence of also burning fat. Another study also claims that CLA might have anti-inflammatory attributes and help the body nullify the growth of tumors (Hubbard et al., 2006). While there's not enough evidence yet to prove it, some scientists and nutritionists believe tallow can also help with absorbing vitamins such as A, D, or K. Assuming this is true, these vitamins play an important role in contributing to a healthy immune system.

Lastly, but as a very important note, tallow has a higher smoke point than most fats and cooking oils, at 480 degrees Fahrenheit. This "smoke point" refers to at what temperature the oil or the fat starts boiling and, with that, starts losing its most important nutrients. So, the higher the smoke point, the greater the chances of using tallow and retaining important nutrients that can be consumed while cooking. To give you an example, the smoke point of canola oil is around 400 degrees Fahrenheit.

While there's more and more evidence that tallow, as a natural animal fat, is a lot healthier than processed seed oils, moderate consumption of tallow is still advised. Also, if using tallow, it's always best to get it from grass-fed cattle instead of the type of tallow most supermarkets seem to sell, where the cattle are fed numerous antibiotics and hormones. Usually, locally bought tallow fits into the healthier category of tallow and is the one that you should strive to purchase. For example, if there are farms nearby, you should try to buy tallow and other animal fats from them rather than from large chain supermarkets.

Butter

As we've previously said, the first traces of humans using butter go back to 8,000 B.C., when a herder walking with a jug filled with warm sheep's milk found out the liquid had solidified with the jostles of the walk, turning it into a delicious paste. However, the beginnings of how butter was created are not 100% certain, since there are reports stating that the earliest evidence of butter only appeared around 2,000 B.C. Either way, butter is one of the first sources of natural fats that humans consumed and incorporated into their diet.

A few years after seed oils first came onto the market, many studies were made to understand the benefits of butter over these oils, and while some of those studies and researchers were inconclusive, many pointed to butter as the healthier option. A study done a few years back reviewed and analyzed the relationship between the consumption of butter and the risk of diabetes, cardiovascular disease, and total mortality, and their conclusion was that the consumption of it had insignificant or neutral associations with any of the health issues analyzed (Pimpin et al., 2016). Because this was a review, the researchers used nine different databases related to butter consumption and cardiovascular issues. Not only that, they had two researchers go through the assessment methods to verify the participants of all the nine studies to understand their characteristics and habits, so this study would be as transparent as possible.

However, much like tallow, nutritionists and doctors recommend organic butter that comes from grass-fed cows. Dr. RJ Burr stated in an article that the recommendation of butter over seed oils is because the latter is heavily processed and the trans fats cause inflammation, as we've reported earlier (Egan, 2016). In the same article, Dr. Meagan Purdy, a naturopathic physician, states that, while butter developed a bad reputation through the 1990s because of the rising popularity of low-fat diets, nutritionists now have a much better understanding that other elements, such as carbohydrates and sugar, are actually the leading cause of obesity, cardiovascular diseases, and diabetes, and not the natural fats found in butter or tallow. However, much like any other fat, moderate consumption of butter is recommended rather than using it in every meal in large proportions.

When talking about butter, it's also important to mention margarine, which is a common replacement for butter, although, as was previously believed, margarine might not be as healthy as some people reported. This is because margarine contains a lot of trans fat, which is bad for your health. In fact, this is backed by a study published in 2015 in the Annals of Epidemiology analyzing the effects of margarine consumption on asthma and allergies in young adults. While the study found no effects of margarine consumption related to allergies, researchers found that the intake of low-fat margarine has a "positive association" with asthma in young adults (Bolte et al., 2005).

When it comes to cooking with butter or seed oils, the experts believe that using butter in moderation when cooking is better because it doesn't turn into toxic chemicals when heated, which can also lead to cardiovascular diseases or cancer (Mendick, 2015).

To give you a more detailed examination of butter and seed oils, we've compared the two on several parameters. While butter has a higher percentage of unsaturated fats than vegetable oil, the latter has higher saturated fats and a longer shelf life, thus having more preservatives, according to Food Struct, a website that compares ingredients and their nutritional values (Yacoubian, 2022). Butter also has more vitamins A and B12, while vegetable oil is richer in vitamins E and K. When it comes to calories, both are high, but vegetable oils contain more when using the same amount, while butter has less fat. Vegetable oil is also devoid of minerals, with the only significant mineral present being iron (around 5%), while butter is richer in minerals, with phosphorus (11%) and calcium (8%) having the highest concentrations. Butter also has more vitamins overall and more diversity in it. Vegetable oil only has vitamins E and K, while butter has vitamins A, E, B12, K, and smaller amounts of B2, B5, and foliate.

Other studies point out that butter can actually decrease pro-inflammatory cytokines and proteins in the body and reduce body weight (Gaullier et al., 2005). Butyrate, often found in butter, can also help with irritable bowel syndrome (IBS) as well as Crohn's disease (Załęski et al., 2013). On the other hand, some vegetable oils, such as corn oil, have been found to increase the chances of cancer in an individual, especially an increase in breast cancer in women, besides all the other negative effects that we've mentioned so far (Moral et al., 2015).

Examination of Coconut, Avocado, and Olive Oil and Their Healthy Benefits

While we've examined healthier alternatives to seed oils such as tallow and butter, there is a group of oils that is generally perceived as being the healthiest there is when it comes to cooking oils and for general consumption. Coconut, olive, or avocado oils are part of those deemed healthy oils, and we will examine them and back our outcomes with research studies.

Coconut Oil

Coconut oil has been used for a long time, with some findings suggesting its use was first documented about 4,000 years ago, not only for consumption but also because of its healing properties. In fact, the coconut is now used in many different industries because of how rich in nutrients it is. Also, most of the coconut can be used for something, from its water, milk, oil, flesh, and fruit. Originally from the regions of the Indian subcontinent, Central America, and South America, the coconut is now consumed and used worldwide.

However, only recently has coconut oil gained popularity in western cuisine. It is said to help with weight loss, improve oral and skin health, and is high in antioxidants. It's also rich in a saturated fat called "medium-chain triglycerides" (MCTs), which studies have proved to have benefits to your health such as weight loss (Mumme & Stonehouse, 2015).

Because of its high MCT content, coconut oil might also be good for fighting infection because of the antifungal and antimicrobial elements found in lauric acid (Hewlings, 2020). This acid is about 50% of the elements found in MCT in coconut oil, which prevents microorganisms such as *Helicobacter pylori* or *Streptococcus mutans* from growing. So, in essence, this oil can also work as a bacteriostatic factor, destroying these bacteria. If you're looking to lose weight, coconut oil, once again because of its MCT elements, might help you by reducing your appetite (Maher & Clegg, 2020). This is because the MCTs you intake break down and create ketones, which are widely known to reduce hunger by limiting your hunger levels through hormones such as ghrelin. The molecules called ketones are the main element in many keto diets that have become extremely popular nowadays.

Speaking of keto diets, it's commonly known that they are great for treating or reducing seizures. While seizures are still a bit of a mystery for researchers, they believe that they are triggered because of a low level of glucose in the brain cells, which helps explain why people tend to have reduced seizures if they follow a keto diet (Crosby et al., 2021). In another recent study published in 2020, researchers tried to find a connection between the keto diet and reducing symptoms of epilepsy, and they found that a slightly altered keto diet with added MCTs and carbs allowed ketosis, and investigators already knew that coconut oil traveled to the human liver where it changed into ketones, helping with epileptic attacks (Morris et al., 2020).

Olive Oil

Olive oil is one of the oldest oils produced by humans, and while there is some uncertainty when it comes to when humans have started to use it, most studies point to the fact that the cultivation of olive trees to produce olive oil started between 4,000 and 2,000 B.C. in Ancient Egypt. Olive oil is considered one of the healthiest oils to use when cooking, especially extra virgin olive oil. Before we continue analyzing the health benefits olive oil has on our body, let's make the distinction between extra virgin olive oil and standard olive oil. Essentially, extra virgin olive oil is the purest type of olive oil we can produce. While when creating standard olive oil, the olive goes through a heating process that allows the separation of the olive and the oil, in the process of making extra virgin olive oil, the only method is pressing, which has to be performed within 72 hours of harvesting the olive. This way of making olive oil makes the product healthier by conserving more nutrients. While extra virgin olive oil tends to be more expensive, you are buying a higher-quality product. Either way, both extra virgin and standard olive oil are known to be healthier than any seed oil.

Olive oil has monounsaturated fats that are extremely healthy. Besides having about 73% of monounsaturated fats, olive oil also has about 11% of polyunsaturated fatty acids and 14% of saturated fat (Cervoni, 2016). Also, one of its components is oleic acid, which has been proven to reduce the growth of cancerous cells as well as inflammation (Menendez & Lupu, 2006). The cause of inflammation is one of the main concerns presented in seed oils; however, olive oil has great anti-inflammatory properties that reduce the chances of metabolic syndrome, obesity, cardiovascular diseases, and even cancer. The anti-inflammatory components presented in olive oil derive from antioxidants such as oleocanthal, which has similar properties to ibuprofen (Lucas et al., 2011). Some researchers believe that oleic acid, which we've already mentioned, might also have anti-inflammatory effects in the body. In a different study, the monounsaturated fat in olive oil has proven to mitigate the risk of strokes along with other cardiovascular issues (Schwingshackl & Hoffmann, 2014).

While heart conditions and heart diseases are the number-one cause of deaths worldwide, they are less prominent in the Mediterranean countries, which is also the part of the world where olive oil is most consumed. There have been numerous researchers looking into the Mediterranean diet to try and understand what ingredients reduce the risks of having these problems. Olive oil, and in particular extra virgin olive oil, is the main ingredient when it comes to reducing heart diseases (R et al., 2013). It helps prevent LDL cholesterol (known as bad cholesterol) from oxidation, lowers blood pressure, and improves the flow in the blood vessels.

Olive oil is also said to be able to fight Alzheimer's disease. This was found after a research study in 2013, where researchers tested oleocanthal from olive oil and found out it dissipated the beta-amyloid in the brain, which helps fight the most common neurodegenerative disease in the world (Abuznait et al., 2013). Alzheimer's disease is caused by tau proteins as well as beta-amyloid accumulation in the brain. Another team of researchers studying the Mediterranean diet reached a similar conclusion. They found out that a Mediterranean-based diet along with extra virgin olive oil or nuts improved cognition, especially when compared to a low-fat diet (Martínez-Lapiscina et al., 2013). As you might know, the Mediterranean diet is a plant-based diet with some meat and fish occasionally but heavily based on vegetables, legumes, whole grains, nuts, seeds, and fruits, where olive oil, especially extra virgin olive oil, is the source of fat. Either way, we will need more research and studies to determine with confidence that there is a relationship between olive oil and the risk of Alzheimer's disease.

The risk of diabetes is one of the main concerns for people who often consume seed oils, but olive oil has proven that it might actually reduce type 2 diabetes. Insulin sensitivity is one of the major causes of type 2 diabetes, since your body is unable to produce insulin. Olive oil brings benefits to blood sugar that affect insulin sensitivity (Kastorini & Panagiotakos, 2009). Many studies have been conducted on the role of olive oil and the Mediterranean diet in lowering the risk of type 2 diabetes, and these studies have included both observational and clinical trials, indicating that there is strong evidence here.

Another advantage of using olive oil is that it has anti-cancer properties. Cancer is one of the most common causes of death anywhere in the world, but as we've pointed out before, the Mediterranean people seem to be less affected by it. Many studies and trials have been conducted by scientists, and many of them point to the antioxidants found in olive oil that prevent cancer growth. In fact, there are studies that clearly show components of olive oil fighting cancer cells in test-tube trials (Menendez et al., 2005). Like many other oleic acid tests, this was conducted in cancer cells of the breast. Either way, the results are quite positive and can potentially translate to other types of cancer. However, we will need more research to make a strong and secure connection between olive oil consumption and the decreased risk of any cancer cells.

The benefits of olive oil to treat rheumatoid arthritis are also well-known and studied. Rheumatoid arthritis is a deformity in the joints and can be quite painful; it is also an autoimmune disease, which is when your body's defenses can't understand the difference between your own body cells and strange cells and so attack yours. Because of its anti-inflammatory characteristics as well as its decrease in oxidative stress, olive oil can bring benefits to people suffering from this problem (L et al., 2014). Researchers have found that to increase the benefits, olive oil can be combined with fish oil because of its high percentage of omega-3 fatty acids (Berbert et al., 2005). In this research, scientists found out that a combination of fish oil and olive oil improved the grip strength dramatically for a patient and helped with morning stiffness in their joints.

While not completely tested, some researchers have shown that olive oil has antibacterial properties. One study in particular has shown that extra virgin olive oil was able to fight eight different strains of bacteria, three of which were resistant to regular antibiotics (Romero et al., 2007). In this particular case, the polyphenol element in olive oil was tested against these bacteria. This study goes even further to state that 30 grams of extra virgin olive oil on a daily basis can decrease the growth of Helicobacter pylori (a bacteria) and eliminate about 40% of it from the human body in only about two to three weeks.

We've seen the differences in processing between standard olive oil and extra virgin, and if you're indecisive, always pick extra virgin olive oil because it's the purest and also retains important nutrients and compounds that standard olive oil doesn't. Another thing to be careful about is some less truthful labels on "extra virgin" olive oils that are often mixed with refined oils. It's always important that you read the labels thoroughly and make sure you're getting extra-virgin olive oil. To summarize, olive oil, particularly extra virgin olive oil, is one of the healthiest oils available. As we've seen, it has benefits for many different aspects of your body and prevents many diseases.

Avocado Oil

The avocado tree is originally from Central America and Mexico, and although most people believe it to be a vegetable, it's actually a fruit. The earliest recordings of the existence of avocados date to around 10,000 B.C., although the signs of human cultivation of the avocado tree suggest around 5,000 B.C. While avocados are originally from Central America, with the Spanish colonization of Central America around the 16th century, the avocado was introduced in Europe and particularly in the Mediterranean regions, which because of their fertile soils allowed the quick adaptation of the avocado tree. From there, it was just a matter of time until it expanded to the rest of the suitable regions of the world.

Avocado is one of the only fruits that is rich in saturated fats that help produce avocado oil, which is not as popular as olive oil but is certainly rising in popularity, mostly because of its health benefits.

To produce avocado oil, the only process that goes through is pressing the pulp of the avocado, and so the majority of the avocado oil components are oleic acid, which we've already seen how beneficial it can be for the body. It also has monounsaturated omega-9 fatty acids, which are considered an extremely healthy fat and are also found in olive oil. The remaining constituents of avocado oil are polyunsaturated fat and saturated fat, which make up a smaller percentage of the elements you get from consuming avocado oil. As we've previously seen, unsaturated fats can be beneficial to reduce both dementia and chronic issues (Flores et al., 2019).

A study wanted to understand how fast the effects of unsaturated fatty acids would appear in the body after a meal using butter and another using avocado oil. In this case, there were about 25 grams of each ingredient, which was 25 grams of unsaturated fat from avocado oil and 25 grams of saturated fat from butter. After only 240 minutes, results started to appear, and the group given the avocado oil-based meal had much lower LDL cholesterol (bad cholesterol), inflammatory cytokines, blood sugar, and triglycerides when compared to the group that had a meal based on butter (Furlan et al., 2017).

Another study did an experiment on rats where one group was given avocado oil and another group was given a blood pressure medication called losartan. In this study, scientists found that the group fed avocado oil had a 21.2% reduction in blood pressure, while the one given losartan had only a 15.5% reduction (Márquez-Ramírez et al., 2018).

The reason oils such as avocado increase certain vitamin absorption is because certain nutrients need to be mixed with healthy fat to be able to be absorbed by the body. This is the case for vitamins such as A, E, D, or K. So, adding avocado oil to your meals will improve the absorption of certain nutrients. Other nutrients, such as beta-carotene and carotenoids usually found in carrots, really need those fats to be absorbed by the body. In a research project, a group of scientists wanted to test exactly that, so they added avocado oil to a salad that included carrots along with other vegetables. They also had a group of participants eat the same salad without the avocado oil, and the results were very interesting, with the salad containing avocado oil having a 17-fold increase in beta-carotene and carotenoids absorption (Unlu et al., 2005).

Comparison of Nutritional Profiles of Seed Oils Vs. Healthy Alternatives

While we've established that the healthier alternatives are better for your health, it's also important to compare them on a nutritional level so you can better understand what you are actually consuming when using these oils. We will compare these three healthier alternatives that we've just talked about—coconut oil, olive oil, and avocado oil—with a generic vegetable oil. Also, the same oils might differ from others, so it's always important that you read the label on them and understand if one brand of healthy oil is better than the other. Also, vegetable oils are mostly made of other oils such as corn, palm, soybean, sunflower, or canola.

Coconut Oil Vs. Vegetable Oil

When looking at minerals, both oils have about 1% of zinc in them, while vegetable oil has 3% more iron than coconut oil, which has about 2% of all the nutrients found in it but also contains more calcium. When it comes to vitamins, vegetable oil has significantly more Vitamin E and K; however, if you remember, healthier oils have healthy fats that allow the absorption of these vitamins a lot more efficiently.

When it comes to the raw data values of nutrients, coconut oil has slightly more calories on average at about 892 kcal per 100 g while vegetable oil has around 884 kcal, but this is a very small difference, and these values might change if you choose another brand.

While both oils are devoid of carbohydrates and proteins, vegetable oil has a higher percentage of fat than coconut oil, and as we've seen, the fat found in vegetable oil is regarded as unhealthy.

Olive Oil Vs. Vegetable Oil

Moving on to olive oil, we start to see even more differences when compared to generic vegetable oil. For one, olive oil is much higher in antioxidants, which have many benefits for your body. Also, it's important to note that because extra virgin olive oil is a lot purer, you will find more healthy nutrients in this version of olive oil. Both vegetable and olive oils contain unsaturated fatty acids; however, olive oil contains oleic acid, which is a monounsaturated fat, as well as palmitic and linoleic acids, while vegetable oil usually only contains omega-6 polyunsaturated fats.

Olive oil also has a much higher percentage of vitamins E and K, which, when added to certain fatty acids such as oleic acid, help the body absorb a lot more of them, while the processing and refining of most seed oils and vegetable oils simply deprives the oil of essential and healthy compounds.

When it comes to fat composition, olive oil has about 73% monounsaturated fats, while generic vegetable oil and seed oil have 62% but also a lower amount of saturated fats (between 6% and 9%) (Diffen, n.d.).

Avocado Oil Vs. Vegetable Oil

Occasionally, avocado oil can also be blended with vegetable oil, but it is far healthier on its own. When comparing avocado oil with generic vegetable oil, the first has far more monounsaturated fat (about 70.5 g per 100 g), while the latter has only about 17.8 g. When it comes to saturated fats, avocado oil has far less—about 11 g against about 26 g—which, in this case, is better, as well as less polyunsaturated fat.

Avocado oil doesn't provide many minerals, while vegetable oil provides a few amounts of zinc and iron. Avocado oil is also far lower in sugar and cholesterol while having essentially the same amount of vitamins and calories. While, overall, both avocado and vegetable have the same amount of fats, the fat in the avocado oil is far more healthier than that found in vegetable oil.

Incorporating Healthy Fats Into Your Diet

Fats are important to consume and to add to your diet. However, the consumption of unhealthy fats from oils such as seed oils can really be dangerous to your health. The use of seed oils is mostly common in frying, and so the single most important tip we can give you when it comes to frying your food is to replace it with a healthy oil, and olive oil is perhaps the best solution because of its great taste. Other healthy oils, such as coconut or avocado oil, are also great choices, but they have a stronger taste that might be a little harder to get used to.

However, besides ditching seed oils completely, there are other ways you can incorporate healthy oils into your body, and some of those don't necessarily require you to use oils at all.

For instance, if you like to have smoothies, yogurt, or cereal for breakfast, one way to introduce healthy fats is to add ground flaxseed, since they are a great source of omega-3 fatty acids. When it comes to dressing your salad, olive oil might be the best choice of all, but avocado oil can also be a great choice. If you're still getting used to the taste of these healthy oils, you can add vinegar along with olive or avocado oil and add it to your salad. In this case, you should skip things like creamy salad dressings since they are a source of unhealthy fats.

If you still feel that your salads need a little kick, you can try tossing some nuts into them, such as crushed walnuts, pumpkin seeds, or even pistachios. Just make sure you check the nutrients in each different nut or seed since these usually vary. Juices, smoothies, or yogurts also go well with some chia seeds.

Chips are a high source of unhealthy fats, but nowadays, you have many different variations, such as chips made of lentils or olives. Because these are still highly processed, we don't recommend having many of them, but they're still a much better choice than classic chips. Finally, eggs are also a great source of healthy fats, and you can eat the whole egg since most of this fat is found in the yolk. The healthiest way to eat eggs is hard-boiled, which you can also add to your salads!

The important thing to remember here is to start changing your habits slowly. If you have been eating unhealthy fats for a long time, it might be hard for your body to adjust to a complete change right away. So, you can start with dressing your salads with healthy oil alternatives, then move on to adding healthy fat to your breakfast, and finally frying with olive oil.

Conclusion

As we've seen through this book, the consumption of seed oils can have negative impacts on your health. While these impacts might vary depending on the seed oil you consume, they all have some negative effects and hardly any benefits. Chronic inflammation is by far the most associated negative effect of seed oils, which is also one of the most common problems in the western population. However, there are other problems that can arise from the consumption of seed oils, such as inflammatory bowel disease, obesity, arthritis, or cardiovascular diseases, mostly because of the imbalance of omega-6 and omega-3 fatty acids.

Besides the tips on how to incorporate healthy oils into your diet, there are other things that will help you reduce or even eliminate seed oils from your diet. For instance, by reading the labels of products you purchase, you can detect products that have seed oil in them or make your own dressing and sauces, such as mayonnaise. Alternatively, if you can't find avocado or olive oil in its purest form, you

Conclusion

can make your own, even if it takes some more work. At least you will know you are eating healthy.

With all of this said and the numerous studies and researchers we've cited, the consumption of seed oils has grown quite a bit over the years, and somehow it's still quite new in the western diet. Because of that, the long-term effects of seed oils are still yet to be discovered. Nevertheless, with the small sample of information we have today, it seems to indicate that seed oils are indeed an unhealthy choice.

Thank you for taking the time to read this book. If you found value in the pages you've just read, it would be greatly appreciated if you could leave a review on Amazon.

Scan this QR code for free future books, free audible codes (when available), and to learn when all of my newest books are released!

Bibliography

Abuznait, A. H., Qosa, H., Busnena, B. A., El Sayed, K. A., & Kaddoumi, A. (2013). Olive-Oil-Derived oleocanthal enhances β-Amyloid clearance as a potential neuroprotective mechanism against alzheimer's disease: In vitro and in vivo studies. ACS Chemical Neuroscience, 4(6), 973–982. https://doi.org/10.1021/cn400024q

Ascherio, A., & Willett, W. C. (1997). Health effects of trans fatty acids. The American Journal of Clinical Nutrition, 66(4), 1006S1010S. https://doi.org/10.1093/ajcn/66.4.1006s

Berbert, A. A., Kondo, C. R. M., Almendra, C. L., Matsuo, T., & Dichi, I. (2005). Supplementation of fish oil and olive oil in patients with rheumatoid arthritis. Nutrition, 21(2), 131–136. https://doi.org/10.1016/j.nut.2004.03.023

Berger, M. E., Smesny, S., Kim, S-W., Davey, C. G., Rice, S., Sarnyai, Z., Schlögelhofer, M., Schäfer, M. R., Berk, M., McGorry, P. D., & Amminger, G. P. (2017). Omega-6 to omega-3 polyunsaturated fatty acid ratio and subsequent mood disorders in young people with at-risk mental states: A 7-year longitudinal study. Translational Psychiatry, 7(8), e1220–e1220. https://doi.org/10.1038/tp.2017.190

Blasbalg, T. L., Hibbeln, J. R., Ramsden, C. E., Majchrzak, S. F., & Rawlings, R. R. (2011). Changes in consumption of omega-3 and omega-6 fatty acids in the united states during the 20th century. The American Journal of Clinical Nutrition, 93(5), 950–962. https://doi.org/10.3945/ajcn.110.006643

Bolte, G., Winkler, G., Hölscher, B., Thefeld, W., Weiland, S. K., & Heinrich, J. (2005). Margarine consumption, asthma, and allergy in young adults: Results of the german national health survey 1998. Annals of Epidemiology, 15(3), 207–213. https://doi.org/10.1016/j.annepidem.2004.04.004

Cervoni, B. (2016, December 22). Olive oil: Nutrition facts. Verywell Fit; Verywell Fit. https://www.verywellfit.com/olive-oil-nutrition-facts-calories-and-health-benefits-4120274

Crosby, L., Davis, B., Joshi, S., Jardine, M., Paul, J., Neola, M., & Barnard, N. D. (2021). Ketogenic diets and chronic disease: Weighing the benefits

Bibliography

against the risks. Frontiers in Nutrition, 8. https://doi.org/10.3389/fnut.2021.702802

Deol, P., Evans, J. R., Dhahbi, J., Chellappa, K., Han, D. S., Spindler, S., & Sladek, F. M. (2015). Soybean oil is more obesogenic and diabetogenic than coconut oil and fructose in mouse: Potential role for the liver. PLOS ONE, 10(7), e0132672. https://doi.org/10.1371/journal.pone.0132672

Diffen. (n.d.). Olive oil vs vegetable oil - difference and comparison | diffen. Diffen. Retrieved January 24, 2023, from https://www.diffen.com/difference/Olive_Oil_vs_Vegetable_Oil

Egan, J. (2016, November 30). Dietary debate: Is oil or butter better for you? The Upside. https://www.vitacost.com/blog/dietary-debate-is-oil-or-butter-better-for-you/.

Flores, M., Saravia, C., Vergara, C., Avila, F., Valdés, H., & Ortiz-Viedma, J. (2019). Avocado oil: Characteristics, properties, and applications. Molecules, 24(11), 2172. https://doi.org/10.3390/molecules24112172

Furlan, C. P. B., Valle, S. C., Östman, E., Maróstica, M. R., & Tovar, J. (2017). Inclusion of hass avocado-oil improves postprandial metabolic responses to a hypercaloric-hyperlipidic meal in overweight subjects. Journal of Functional Foods, 38, 349–354. https://doi.org/10.1016/j.jff.2017.09.019

Gaullier, J.-M., Halse, J., Høye, K., Kristiansen, K., Fagertun, H., Vik, H., & Gudmundsen, O. (2005). Supplementation with conjugated linoleic acid for 24 months is well tolerated by and reduces body fat mass in healthy, overweight humans. The Journal of Nutrition, 135(4), 778–784. https://doi.org/10.1093/jn/135.4.778

Gunnars, K. (2018). Top 10 evidence-based health benefits of coconut oil. Healthline. https://www.healthline.com/nutrition/top-10-evidence-based-health-benefits-of-coconut-oil

Heileson, J. L. (2019). Dietary saturated fat and heart disease: A narrative review. Nutrition Reviews, 78(6). https://doi.org/10.1093/nutrit/nuz091

Hewlings, S. (2020). Coconuts and health: Different chain lengths of saturated fats require different consideration. Journal of Cardiovascular Development and Disease, 7(4), 59. https://doi.org/10.3390/jcdd7040059

History Cooperative. (2019, January 10). The history and origins of avocado oil. History Cooperative. https://historycooperative.org/history-of-avocado-oil/

Horstman, E. (2022, April 9). Sneaky industrial seed oils are making us sick.

Bibliography

Camille Styles. https://camillestyles.com/wellness/industrial-seed-oils/

Hubbard, N. E., Lim, D., & Erickson, K. L. (2006). Beef tallow increases the potency of conjugated linoleic acid in the reduction of mouse mammary tumor metastasis. The Journal of Nutrition, 136(1), 88–93. https://doi.org/10.1093/jn/136.1.88

Kastorini, C.-M., & Panagiotakos, D. (2009). Dietary patterns and prevention of type 2 diabetes: From research to clinical practice; A systematic review. Current Diabetes Reviews, 5(4), 221–227. https://doi.org/10.2174/157339909789804341

Kutilek, P. (2022, June 15). Olive oil versus extra virgin olive oil: What's the difference? Dinner Kits Designed for 15 Minutes with 1 Pan | Gobble. https://www.gobble.com/blog/olive-oil-vs-extra-virgin-olive-oil/

L, G. C., B, R.-R., & L, C.-C. (2014, February 1). [Importance of nutritional treatment in the inflammatory process of rheumatoid arthritis patients; A review]. Nutricion Hospitalaria. https://pubmed.ncbi.nlm.nih.gov/24528339/

Lauretti, E., & Praticò, D. (2017). Effect of canola oil consumption on memory, synapse and neuropathology in the triple transgenic mouse model of alzheimer's disease. Scientific Reports, 7(1). https://doi.org/10.1038/s41598-017-17373-3

Leech, J. (2018, September 14). 11 proven benefits of olive oil. Healthline. https://www.healthline.com/nutrition/11-proven-benefits-of-olive-oil#TOC_TITLE_HDR_14

Levy, J. (2020, June 27). Can you eat tallow? 5 reasons to use this form of fat. Dr. Axe. https://draxe.com/nutrition/tallow/

Lucas, L., Russell, A., & Keast, R. (2011). Molecular mechanisms of inflammation. anti-inflammatory benefits of virgin olive oil and the phenolic compound oleocanthal. Current Pharmaceutical Design, 17(8), 754–768. https://doi.org/10.2174/138161211795428911

Maher, T., & Clegg, M. E. (2020). A systematic review and meta-analysis of medium-chain triglycerides effects on acute satiety and food intake. Critical Reviews in Food Science and Nutrition, 1–13. https://doi.org/10.1080/10408398.2020.1742654

Mancini, A., Imperlini, E., Nigro, E., Montagnese, C., Daniele, A., Orrù, S., & Buono, P. (2015). Biological and nutritional properties of palm oil and palmitic acid: Effects on health. Molecules, 20(9), 17339–17361. https://doi.org/10.3390/molecules200917339

Márquez-Ramírez, C. A., Hernández de la Paz, J. L., Ortiz-Avila, O., Raya-Farias, A., González-Hernández, J. C., Rodríguez-Orozco, A. R., Salgado-Garciglia, R., Saavedra-Molina, A., Godínez-Hernández, D., &

Bibliography

Cortés-Rojo, C. (2018). Comparative effects of avocado oil and losartan on blood pressure, renal vascular function, and mitochondrial oxidative stress in hypertensive rats. Nutrition, 54, 60–67. https://doi.org/10.1016/j.nut.2018.02.024

Martínez-Lapiscina, E. H., Clavero, P., Toledo, E., Estruch, R., Salas-Salvadó, J., San Julián, B., Sanchez-Tainta, A., Ros, E., Valls-Pedret, C., & Martinez-Gonzalez, M. Á. (2013). Mediterranean diet improves cognition: The PREDIMED-NAVARRA randomised trial. Journal of Neurology, Neurosurgery & Psychiatry, 84(12), 1318–1325. https://doi.org/10.1136/jnnp-2012-304792

Masi, L. N., Martins, A. R., Neto, J. C. R., Amaral, C. L. do, Crisma, A. R., Vinolo, M. A. R., de Lima Júnior, E. A., Hirabara, S. M., & Curi, R. (2012). Sunflower oil supplementation has proinflammatory effects and does not reverse insulin resistance in obesity induced by high-fat diet in C57BL/6 mice. Journal of Biomedicine and Biotechnology, 2012, 1–9. https://doi.org/10.1155/2012/945131

Mendick, R. (2015, November 7). Cooking with vegetable oils releases toxic cancer-causing chemicals, say experts. Telegraph.co.uk. https://www.telegraph.co.uk/news/health/news/11981884/Cooking-with-vegetable-oils-releases-toxic-cancer-causing-chemicals-say-experts.html

Menendez, J. A., Vellon, L., Colomer, R., & Lupu, R. (2005). Oleic acid, the main monounsaturated fatty acid of olive oil, suppresses her-2/neu (erbb-2) expression and synergistically enhances the growth inhibitory effects of trastuzumab (herceptin^{TM}) in breast cancer cells with her-2/neu oncogene amplification. Annals of Oncology, 16(3), 359–371. https://doi.org/10.1093/annonc/mdi090

Menendez, J., & Lupu, R. (2006). Mediterranean dietary traditions for the molecular treatment of human cancer: Anti-Oncogenic actions of the main olive oils monounsaturated fatty acid oleic acid. Current Pharmaceutical Biotechnology, 7(6), 495–502. https://doi.org/10.2174/138920106779116900

Messina, M., Shearer, G., & Petersen, K. (2021). Soybean oil lowers circulating cholesterol levels and coronary heart disease risk, and has no effect on markers of inflammation and oxidation. Nutrition, 111343. https://doi.org/10.1016/j.nut.2021.111343

Moral, R., Escrich, R., Solanas, M., Vela, E., Ruiz de Villa, M. C., & Escrich, E. (2015). Diets high in corn oil or extra-virgin olive oil differentially modify the gene expression profile of the mammary gland and influence

Bibliography

experimental breast cancer susceptibility. European Journal of Nutrition, 55(4), 1397–1409. https://doi.org/10.1007/s00394-015-0958-2

Morris, G., Maes, M., Berk, M., Carvalho, A. F., & Puri, B. K. (2020). Nutritional ketosis as an intervention to relieve astrogliosis: Possible therapeutic applications in the treatment of neurodegenerative and neuroprogressive disorders. European Psychiatry, 63(1). https://doi.org/10.1192/j.eurpsy.2019.13

Mu, H., Wei, C., Xu, W., Gao, W., Zhang, W., & Mai, K. (2020). Effects of replacement of dietary fish oil by rapeseed oil on growth performance, anti-oxidative capacity and inflammatory response in large yellow croaker larimichthys crocea. Aquaculture Reports, 16, 100251. https://doi.org/10.1016/j.aqrep.2019.100251

Mumme, K., & Stonehouse, W. (2015). Effects of medium-chain triglycerides on weight loss and body composition: A meta-analysis of randomized controlled trials. Journal of the Academy of Nutrition and Dietetics, 115(2), 249–263. https://doi.org/10.1016/j.jand.2014.10.022

Nast, C. (2021, October 14). Seed Oil Is the Latest Thing We're Being Told to Eliminate from Our Diets—Here's Why. GQ. https://www.gq.com/story/seed-oil-health

Nobuyuki Ito, Masao Hirose, Akihiro Hagiwara, & Satoru Takahashi. (2020). Carcinogenicity and modification of carcinogenic response by antioxidants. SpringerLink, 52, 183–194. https://doi.org/10.1007/978-1-4615-9561-8_15

Oteng, A.-B., & Kersten, S. (2019). Mechanisms of action of trans fatty acids. Advances in Nutrition, 11(3). https://doi.org/10.1093/advances/nmz125

Ouilly, J. T., Bazongo, P., Bougma, A., Kaboré, N., Lykke, A. M., Ouédraogo, A., & Bassolé, I. H. N. (2017). Chemical composition, physicochemical characteristics, and nutritional value of lannea kerstingii seeds and seed oil. Journal of Analytical Methods in Chemistry, 2017, 1–6. https://doi.org/10.1155/2017/2840718

Pimpin, L., Wu, J. H. Y., Haskelberg, H., Del Gobbo, L., & Mozaffarian, D. (2016). Is butter back? A systematic review and meta-analysis of butter consumption and risk of cardiovascular disease, diabetes, and total mortality. PLOS ONE, 11(6), e0158118. https://doi.org/10.1371/journal.pone.0158118

R, E., E, R., J, S.-S., Mi, C., D, C., F, A., E, G.-G., V, R.-G., M, F., J, L., Rm, L.-R., L, S.-M., X, P., J, B., Ma, M., Jv, S., Ja, M., & Ma, M.-G. (2013, April 4). Primary prevention of cardiovascular disease with a mediter-

Bibliography

ranean diet. The New England Journal of Medicine. https://pubmed.ncbi.nlm.nih.gov/23432189/

Ramsden, C. E., Faurot, K. R., Carrera-Bastos, P., Cordain, L., De Lorgeril, M., & Sperling, L. S. (2009). Dietary fat quality and coronary heart disease prevention: A unified theory based on evolutionary, historical, global, and modern perspectives. Current Treatment Options in Cardiovascular Medicine, 11(4), 289–301. https://doi.org/10.1007/s11936-009-0030-8

Romero, C., Medina, E., Vargas, J., Brenes, M., & De Castro, A. (2007). In vitro activity of olive oil polyphenols against helicobacter pylori. Journal of Agricultural and Food Chemistry, 55(3), 680–686. https://doi.org/10.1021/jf0630217

Schwingshackl, L., & Hoffmann, G. (2014). Monounsaturated fatty acids, olive oil and health status: A systematic review and meta-analysis of cohort studies. Lipids in Health and Disease, 13(1). https://doi.org/10.1186/1476-511x-13-154

Simson, R. (n.d.). 10 tips for incorporating healthy fats into your diet. Roswell Park Comprehensive Cancer Center. https://www.roswellpark.org/cancertalk/201706/10-tips-incorporating-healthy-fats-your-diet

Sun, Y., Magnussen, C. G., Dwyer, T., Oddy, W. H., Venn, A. J., & Smith, K. J. (2018). Cross-Sectional associations between dietary fat-related behaviors and continuous metabolic syndrome score among young australian adults. Nutrients, 10(8), 972. https://doi.org/10.3390/nu10080972

Takeda, M., Imaizumi, M., Sawano, S., Manabe, Y., & Fushiki, T. (2001). Long-term optional ingestion of corn oil induces excessive caloric intake and obesity in mice. Nutrition, 17(2), 117–120. https://doi.org/10.1016/s0899-9007(00)00513-x

Unlu, N. Z., Bohn, T., Clinton, S. K., & Schwartz, S. J. (2005). Carotenoid absorption from salad and salsa by humans is enhanced by the addition of avocado or avocado oil. The Journal of Nutrition, 135(3), 431–436. https://doi.org/10.1093/jn/135.3.431

US Department of Agriculture. (n.d.). FoodData central. Fdc.nal.usda.gov. https://fdc.nal.usda.gov/fdc-app.html#/food-details/171400/nutrients

USDA. (n.d.). Oil crops sector at a glance. Ers.usda.gov. https://www.ers.usda.gov/topics/crops/soybeans-and-oil-crops/oil-crops-sector-at-a-glance/

WebMD Editorial Contributors. (2022, November 28). Sunflower oil: Is it good for you? WebMD. https://www.webmd.com/diet/sunflower-oil-good-for-you

Bibliography

Wendell, S. G., Baffi, C., & Holguin, F. (2014). Fatty acids, inflammation, and asthma. Journal of Allergy and Clinical Immunology, 133(5), 1255–1264. https://doi.org/10.1016/j.jaci.2013.12.1087

Whigham, L. D., Watras, A. C., & Schoeller, D. A. (2007). Efficacy of conjugated linoleic acid for reducing fat mass: A meta-analysis in humans. The American Journal of Clinical Nutrition, 85(5), 1203–1211. https://doi.org/10.1093/ajcn/85.5.1203

Yacoubian, J. (2022, March 10). Vegetable oil vs butter - health impact and nutrition comparison. Food Struct. https://foodstruct.com/compare/vegetable-oil-vs-butter

Załęski, A., Banaszkiewicz, A., & Walkowiak, J. (2013). Butyric acid in irritable bowel syndrome. Gastroenterology Review, 6, 350–353. https://doi.org/10.5114/pg.2013.39917

Printed in Great Britain
by Amazon